Psychological first aid
during Ebola virus disease outbreaks

PFA GUIDE

FOREWORD

Ebola virus disease outbreaks have a significant impact on the wellbeing of those affected, their family, community members and the health workers treating people with Ebola.

This guide focuses on **psychological first aid**, which involves humane, supportive and practical help to fellow human beings suffering serious crisis events. It is written for people who can help others experiencing an extremely distressing event.

This guide is an adaptation of the *Psychological first aid: Guide for field workers (World Health Organization, War Trauma Foundation, World Vision International, 2011)*. It has been adapted to better respond to the challenges of Ebola virus disease outbreaks. Ebola poses specific problems for affected people (e.g., stigmatization, isolation, fear, and possible abandonment), their caregivers and responders (e.g., safety, access to updated information).

Psychological first aid has been recommended by many expert groups, including the Inter-Agency Standing Committee (IASC) and the Sphere Project. In 2009, the World Health Organization's (WHO) mental health Gap Action Programme (mhGAP) Guideline Development Group evaluated the evidence for psychological first aid and psychological debriefing. It concluded that psychological first aid, rather than psychological debriefing, should be offered to people in severe distress following recent exposure to a traumatic event.

Endorsed by many international agencies, the original Psychological First Aid Guide reflects the emerging science and international consensus on how to support people in the immediate aftermath of extremely stressful events.

CONTENTS

INTRODUCTION UNDERSTANDING EBOLA VIRUS DISEASE		4
CHAPTER 1 UNDERSTANDING PSYCHOLOGICAL FIRST AID		12
1.1	How do crisis events affect people?	13
1.2	What is Psychological First Aid?	14
1.3	Psychological First Aid: who, when and where?	15
CHAPTER 2 HOW TO HELP RESPONSIBLY		20
2.1	Respect safety, dignity and rights	21
2.2	Be aware of other available emergency response measures	23
2.3	Look after yourself	23
CHAPTER 3 PROVIDING PSYCHOLOGICAL FIRST AID		24
3.1	Good communication with people in distress	25
3.2	Preparing to help	27
3.3	The Action Principles of PFA: Look, Listen and Link!	28
3.4	People who likely need special attention	40
CHAPTER 4 CARING FOR YOURSELF AND YOUR COLLEAGUES		46
4.1	Getting ready to help	47
4.2	Managing stress: Healthy work and life habits	48
4.3	Rest and reflection	49

OFFERING PSYCHOLOGICAL FIRST AID TO GRIEVING PEOPLE	50
RELAXATION AND BREATHING EXERCISES	52
CONTACT LIST OF MENTAL HEALTH AND PSYCHOSOCIAL RESOURCES IN YOUR AREA	54
LOCAL ALTERNATIVE RITUALS FOR SAFE MOURNING AFTER THE DEATH OF A PERSON WITH EBOLA	55
PSYCHOLOGICAL FIRST AID: POCKET GUIDE	56
CONTACT LIST OF EBOLA DISEASE OUTBREAK SERVICES IN YOUR AREA	**BACK COVER**

INTRODUCTION
UNDERSTANDING EBOLA VIRUS DISEASE

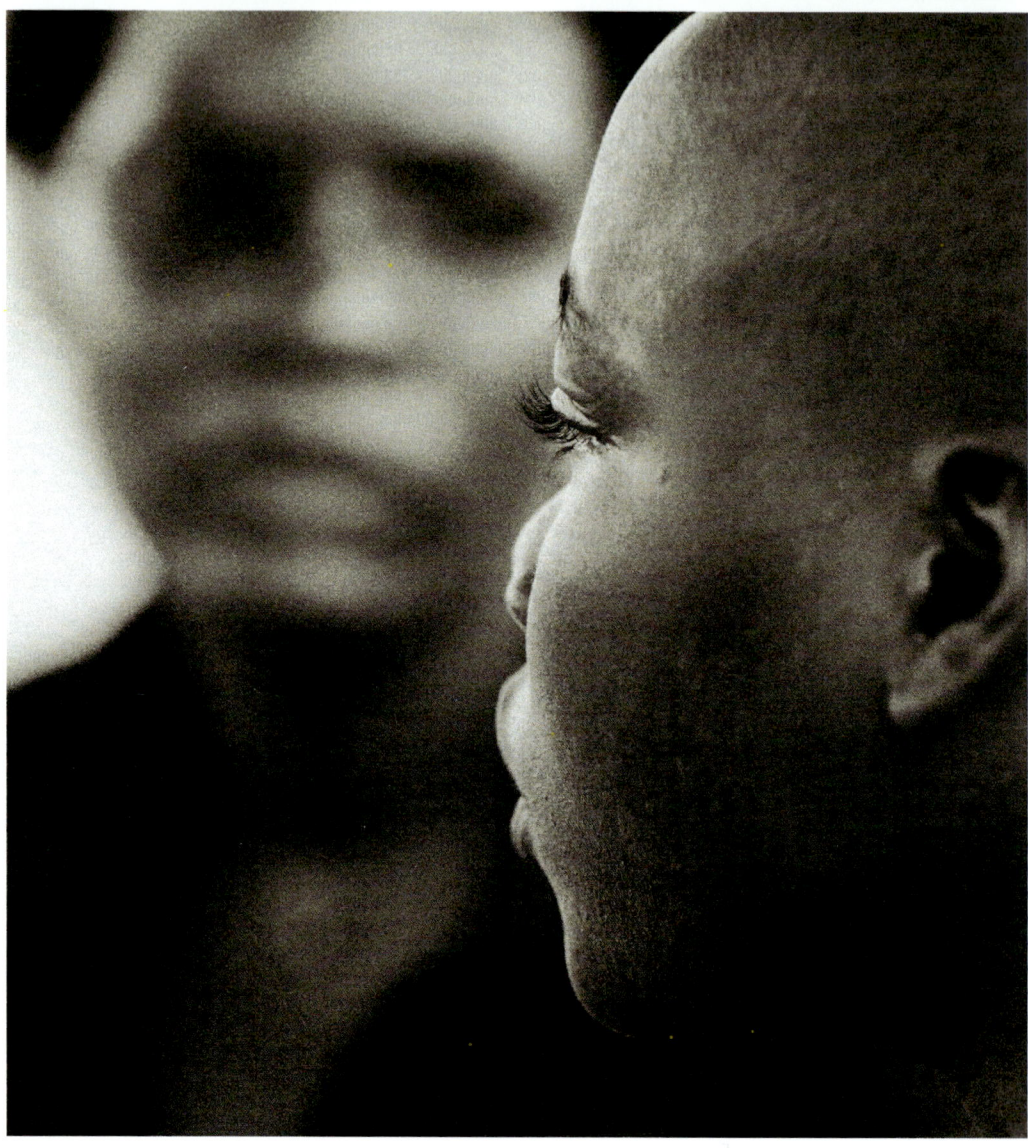

IN THIS CHAPTER WE DISCUSS:

- A   WHAT IS EBOLA VIRUS DISEASE?
- B   HOW DOES IT SPREAD?
- C   HOW CAN IT BE PREVENTED?

A   WHAT IS EBOLA VIRUS DISEASE?

Ebola virus disease is a severe, infectious disease that can be fatal (the case fatality rate of the 2014 outbreak in West Africa is about 50%). However, health care substantially increases a person's chance of survival.

Appropriate infection prevention and control measures in treatment centres and hospitals, at community gatherings, during burial ceremonies and at home can help reduce the spread of the disease. You can protect yourself, your family and your community by following the advice on these measures below.

WHO IS AT RISK OF EBOLA VIRUS DISEASE?

A person is at risk if they have:

- »   spent time with someone sick with Ebola or;
- »   attended a funeral of someone who has recently died with symptoms of Ebola.

SIGNS, SYMPTOMS AND COURSE OF ILLNESS

> **Ebola starts suddenly with a high fever. A person with Ebola feels very tired, has a headache and aches in the body, and does not want to eat. The time from infection with the virus to the onset of symptoms is 2 to 21 days.**

The person with the Ebola virus can infect others as soon as they begin to have symptoms.

Early-stage Ebola disease may be confused with other infectious diseases (e.g., malaria) because the initial symptoms are nonspecific. These symptoms include a high fever and extreme tiredness, often accompanied by appetite loss, headache, and body pain.

As the disease progresses, people begin to experience vomiting and diarrhoea.

Blood in vomit or stool is seen among severely ill patients, mostly in **later stages**, and is often followed by death within days.

In non-fatal cases, the person may improve around days 6-11 and will no longer be infectious.

ADVICE FOR INDIVIDUALS AND FAMILIES IN EBOLA-AFFECTED AREAS

WHAT SHOULD I DO?

CALL FOR HELP IMMEDIATELY
Early treatment increases the chance of survival for the person, and prevents the spread of disease to others.

- If you suspect a family member or someone in the community of having Ebola, encourage and support them in seeking appropriate medical attention in an Ebola Treatment Centre.
- If they cannot go to the treatment centre, hospital or health post for any reason, you should speak with your local community leader immediately or call the Ebola Hotline for help. Health care workers or anyone who transports sick people to treatment centres should use **personal protective equipment** and observe infection prevention and control measures. Personal protective equipment includes heavy clothing, gloves, goggles and masks.
- If someone in your community has recovered from Ebola, ask this person to help. As far as is known, once a person has recovered from Ebola, they have immunity against the virus.

WHILE YOU ARE WAITING FOR HELP YOU SHOULD:

PROTECT YOUR FAMILY

- Provide the sick person with their own space, separate from the rest of the family. Provide them with their own plate, cup, cutlery (e.g., spoon, fork), toothbrush, etc. No item should be shared with others.
- Only one family or community member should care for the sick person. Others should not come into contact with them.
- Avoid touching the sick person. All body fluids including stool, vomit, blood, breast milk, sperm, urine and sweat are dangerous and must not be touched. If you need to touch, you must wear gloves. Make sure the gloves have no holes. You can get gloves from community helpers and health posts or from a shop. Put soiled (dirty) clothes, towels and bed linen in a plastic bag and incinerate (burn them).
- A person with Ebola is best cared for in a hospital or Ebola treatment centre. However, if you provide extended care for a person with Ebola in your home you will need personal protective equipment. Ask your local health post to provide this. WHO does not recommend caring for a person with Ebola at home.
- Wash hands with soap and water or rub hands with an alcohol-based hand sanitizer (community workers may be able to provide this):
    - after touching the sick person or anything that belongs to the person;
    - after touching a used toilet;
    - after touching any blood or body fluids (e.g., faeces, vomit);
    - after touching anything that could be contaminated with body fluids, **even if you wore gloves**; and
    - after removing gloves.

CARE FOR THE SICK

» Provide plenty of drinks for the sick person such as water, soup, tea or locally available beverages. If possible, encourage the sick person to feed little by little, "spoon by spoon".
» Give paracetamol to the person, if they are suffering from fever and pain. Do not give aspirin or any other pain killer.

DANGER SIGNS

If the patient vomits, has diarrhoea or starts to bleed, they must be transported to a hospital immediately. **These are the danger signs.** The patient can **infect others** and is at **risk of dying**.

The patient should be moved only by health workers who have **personal protective equipment** under the guidance of local authorities.

B HOW DOES EBOLA VIRUS DISEASE SPREAD AND HOW CAN IT BE PREVENTED?

Unlike infections such as influenza or tuberculosis, Ebola is not airborne. It can be spread only by direct contact with the body fluids or tissues of a person who is sick with the disease or who has died, or by contact with anything the sick or dead person has used or touched, such as soiled (dirty) linen and clothing.

Ebola is spread through:

- direct contact with an affected person's wounds, tissues, and body fluids like stool, vomit, blood, breast milk, sperm, urine and sweat. These are dangerous and must not be touched;
- contact with an infected person's soiled (dirty) clothing or bed linen;
- unsterilized injections;
- skin piercing instruments (e.g., syringes or needles) that have been used by an infected person;
- direct physical handling of persons who have died of Ebola.

Since Ebola spreads through direct contact with an infected person, those living with and caring for a person with Ebola are at high risk of infection. Personal protective equipment should be used when caring for a patient at home. Appropriate infection prevention and control measures are crucial to reduce the risk of infection.

People with symptoms should avoid all physical contact with others.

Protect yourself after someone has died of Ebola: avoid direct contact and implement protective measures

» People who have died of Ebola are still infectious, and people in direct contact with their bodies are at risk. **Do not touch or move** the body of someone who has died of Ebola. Dead bodies should be handled only by people appropriately trained and wearing personal protective equipment.
» During funerals and burial rituals, **do not touch** the bodies of the deceased. See page 55 for ideas about how to safely mourn and honour the deceased person.
» Wear gloves when touching a dead person's soiled clothes, towels and bed linen, and put them in a plastic bag and incinerate (burn them). It will prevent you from getting infected.

Information for those who have fully recovered from Ebola

Health care providers should closely monitor people recovering from Ebola, ideally using laboratory tests, to be sure that the virus is no longer in the person's system. Keep in mind the following information about people who have recovered from Ebola:

» As far as is known, the person has immunity against Ebola disease.
» The person can no longer infect others.
» The person can help the community by taking care of sick people.
» Men who recover from Ebola should wear a condom during sexual contact for at least 3 months after recovery – Ebola is present in the semen up to this time.
» Before breastfeeding, the breast milk of women who have recovered from Ebola should be laboratory tested.

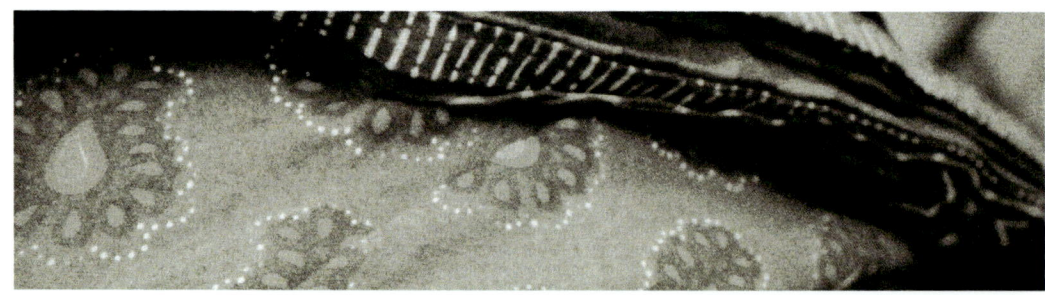

CHAPTER 1
UNDERSTANDING PSYCHOLOGICAL FIRST AID

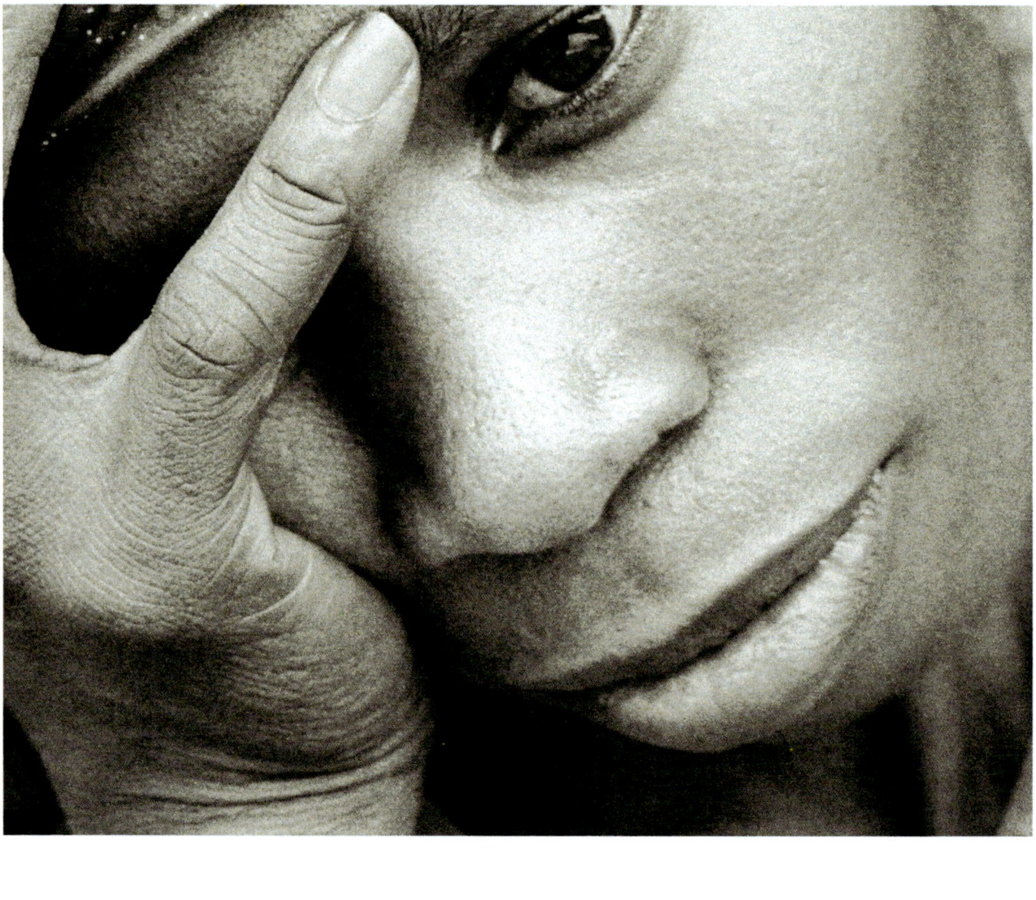

IN THIS CHAPTER WE DISCUSS:

1.1 HOW DO CRISIS EVENTS AFFECT PEOPLE?
1.2 WHAT IS PSYCHOLOGICAL FIRST AID?
1.3 PFA: WHO, WHEN AND WHERE?

1.1 HOW DO CRISIS EVENTS AFFECT PEOPLE?

Communities can be severely affected by Ebola disease in many ways. People are separated from their loved ones, due to illness or death. Health workers need to deal with a high workload and a lot of stress. Those associated with Ebola can be vulnerable to social stigma, worsening their distress and isolation. Ultimately, whole communities may experience the fear and suffering that disease outbreaks often cause.

Although these events affect everyone in some way, people can experience a wide range of reactions. They can feel overwhelmed, confused or very uncertain about what is happening. They can feel fearful and anxious, or numb and detached. Some people may have mild reactions, whereas others may have more severe reactions. In general, how someone reacts depends on many factors, including:

» the nature and severity of the event;
» their experience with previous distressing events;
» the support they have in their life from others;
» their physical health;
» their personal and family history of mental health problems;
» their cultural background and traditions;
» their age (for example, children of different age groups react differently).

It is also important to remember that Ebola influences how we normally provide support to each other (e.g., by not being able to touch people) and how we cope with the death of our loved ones (e.g., by not being able to engage in traditional burials). This can severely worsen people's distress.

Every person has strengths and abilities to help them cope with life's challenges. However, some people are particularly vulnerable in a crisis situation and may need extra help. This includes people who may be at risk of being infected, such as those who have been in contact with someone sick with symptoms of Ebola (e.g., health care providers) or people who have attended the funeral of someone who has recently died of Ebola (e.g., relatives of people with Ebola). Other vulnerable people may include those who need additional support because of their age (children and the elderly), because they have a mental or physical disability, or because they belong to marginalized groups (including migrants). Children whose parents died of the disease, and Ebola survivors, may be stigmatised and rejected by their communities. Therefore, they may not receive the support they need.

See section 3.4 for guidance in helping vulnerable people.

1.2 WHAT IS PSYCHOLOGICAL FIRST AID?

According to the Sphere Project (2011) and IASC (2007), Psychological First Aid (PFA) describes *a humane, supportive response to someone who is suffering and may need support.* PFA involves:

- providing non-intrusive, practical care and support;
- assessing needs and concerns;
- helping people to address basic needs (food and water, information);
- listening to people, but not pressuring them to talk;
- comforting people and helping them to feel calm;
- helping people connect to information, services and social supports;
  - In the case of Ebola disease, information is vital: those providing PFA can help to dispel myths, share clear messages about healthy behaviour and improve people's understanding of the disease;
- protecting people from further harm (see also section 3.4 on people who likely need special attention).

IT IS ALSO IMPORTANT TO UNDERSTAND WHAT PFA IS NOT:

- » It is not something that only professionals can do.
- » It is not professional counselling.
- » It does not necessarily involve a detailed discussion of the event that caused the distress (as in "psychological debriefing"[1]).
- » It is not asking someone to analyse what happened to them or to put time and events in order.
- » It is not about pressuring people to tell you their feelings and reactions to an event, but rather being available to listen to people.

Overall, PFA involves helping people to:

- » feel safe, connected to others, calm and hopeful;
- » have access to social, physical and emotional support; and
- » feel able to help themselves, as individuals and communities.

---

[1] *WHO (2010) and Sphere (2011) describe psychological debriefing as promoting ventilation by asking a person to briefly but systematically recount their perceptions, thoughts and emotional reactions during a recent stressful event. This intervention is not recommended. This is distinct from routine operational debriefing of aid workers used by some organizations at the end of a mission or work task.*

1.3 PSYCHOLOGICAL FIRST AID: WHO, WHEN AND WHERE?

WHO CAN BENEFIT FROM PFA?

PFA is for distressed people recently exposed to a crisis event. You can help both children and adults, although not everyone who experiences a crisis event will need or want PFA. **Do not force** help onto people, but make yourself easily available to those who may want support.

People who may benefit from PFA during an Ebola outbreak include distressed health care providers treating people with Ebola, members of the community feeling anxious about infection, or people experiencing distress even though they have received confirmation that they do not have Ebola.

However, there may be situations when someone needs much more advanced mental health support. When providing PFA during a disease outbreak, it is especially important to help people who have been exposed to the disease and/or have symptoms to access immediate medical attention. **Know your limits** and get help from others, such as health personnel (including, where relevant and available, mental health nurses and clinicians in district hospitals), your colleagues, local authorities, or community and religious leaders.

People who need more than PFA in terms of mental health support include:

- people who are so upset that they cannot care for themselves or their children;
- people at risk of hurting themselves;
- people at risk of hurting others.

You may also encounter people suffering in other ways as a consequence of the Ebola disease outbreak. You can offer PFA and determine if they may need further specialized support. This may include people who have lost multiple family members and loved ones to Ebola, particularly orphans who need extra care and protection. PFA may also be useful for people who may be stigmatized by their communities, such as:

- people who have recovered from Ebola;
- health care providers treating people with Ebola;
- frontline workers of Ebola operations (e.g., people involved in dead body management).

WHEN IS PFA PROVIDED?

Although people may need access to help and support for a long time after an event, PFA is aimed at helping people who have been very recently affected by a crisis event. You can provide PFA when you first have contact with very distressed people. This is usually during or immediately after an event. However, it may sometimes be days or weeks after, depending on how long the event lasted and how severe it was.

During the Ebola outbreak, for example, PFA can be offered:

» during contact tracing of people who have had contact with a person with Ebola;
» when delivering survival and hygiene kits to people who recovered but whose properties (e.g., clothing and bedding) were destroyed during disinfection of their home;
» when supporting a health care provider experiencing distress after a long shift at a clinic;
» when supporting a family or community that has lost someone to Ebola and is suffering because their loved one cannot be buried according to tradition;
» when supporting a child whose parents are in hospital, and who may be feeling confused and sad (see section 3.4 for further advice on supporting separated children and adolescents);
» when helping members of the community share their frustrations about travel restrictions.

WHERE IS PFA PROVIDED?

You can offer PFA wherever it is safe enough to do so. This is often in

- » community settings;
- » places where distressed people are assisted, such as health centres, shelters or camps, and schools.

In the case of an Ebola (or other contagious disease) outbreak, **safety from exposure to the disease** is the most important consideration in where to offer PFA – for yourself, the person and others. This means taking all relevant precautions to prevent infection, and ensuring that the appropriate medical care is offered immediately to people who have symptoms.

When providing PFA, it is essential to respect a person's confidentiality and dignity. Ideally, try to provide PFA where you can have some privacy to talk with the person, when appropriate and possible, while still adhering to safety precautions. This is important not only for confidentiality, but also to avoid the spread of panic or rumours in the community.

However, during disease outbreaks, there are limits to confidentiality because of the importance of stopping the spread of the disease. Explain to the person that personal matters shared with you will be kept confidential, but you are required to report to health surveillance teams if the person may have been exposed to Ebola and/or has symptoms of the disease. Also, some families do not want to give up the body of a loved one who has died at home to health teams for burial. They may not understand the serious risk of infection for others in the house.

Be gentle as you talk with people and acknowledge their fears or concerns. Explain in ways they can understand the importance of informing the authorities of suspected cases of Ebola – to promote the health and safety of the person, their family and their community. You can tell them that:

- » early detection and supportive treatments improve the chance of survival;
- » going to hospital to find out their disease status can help protect their family and the community from infection;
- » there is a high risk of infection for anyone in the house who comes in contact with a dead person's body;
- » there may be support measures available from the government to help people recovering from the illness (e.g., government assistance and material items and services given when a person is discharged from hospital).

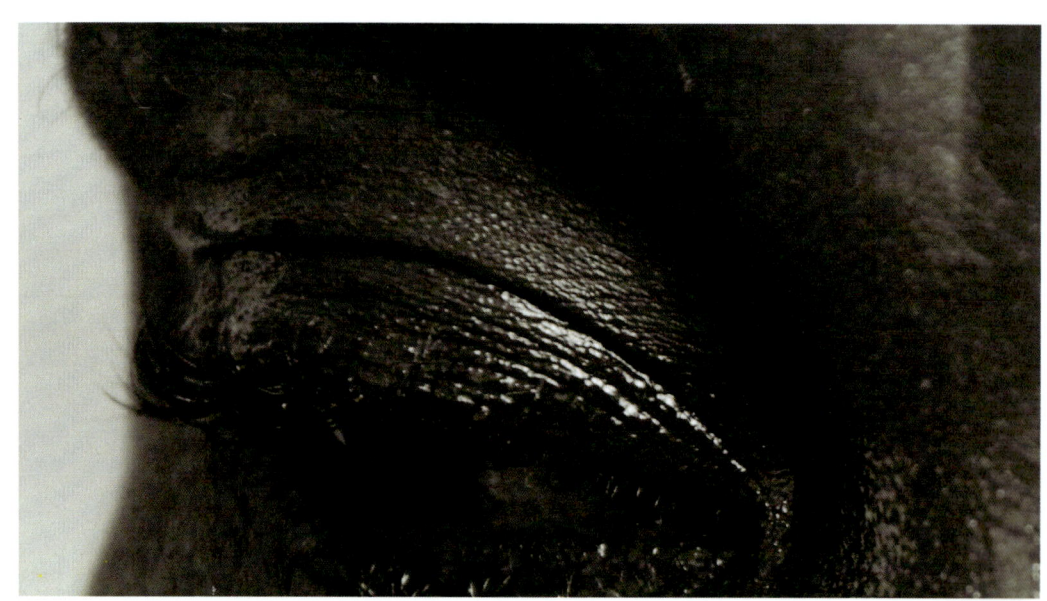

CHAPTER 2
HOW TO HELP RESPONSIBLY

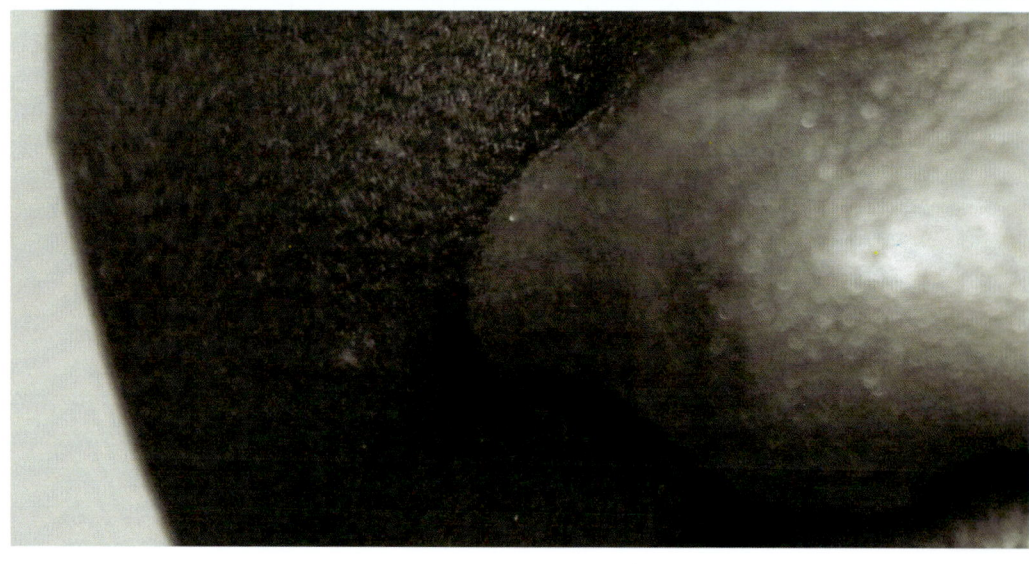

HELPING RESPONSIBLY INVOLVES THREE MAIN POINTS:

2.1 RESPECT SAFETY, DIGNITY AND RIGHTS
2.2 BE AWARE OF OTHER EMERGENCY RESPONSE MEASURES
2.3 LOOK AFTER YOURSELF

2.1 RESPECT SAFETY, DIGNITY AND RIGHTS

When you take on the responsibility of helping people affected by a distressing event, it is important to respect their safety, dignity and rights. The following principles apply to any person or agency involved in a humanitarian response, including those providing PFA during disease outbreaks.

RESPECT PEOPLE'S:

Safety:

- » Avoid putting people at further risk of harm as a result of your actions.
    - » For example, avoid putting them at risk of infection by taking all necessary safety precautions.
- » Make sure, to the best of your ability, that the adults and children you help are safe and protect them from physical or psychological harm.
    - » For example, many Ebola survivors are discriminated against. Do not expose them to further stigma. Instead, encourage them to think about how they can help others if they can and are willing, by perhaps taking care of sick relatives.

Dignity

- » Treat all people with respect. The situation in areas affected by the Ebola disease outbreak will be challenging for everybody. Fear, grief and tension are likely to increase in the community. In these difficult moments, more than ever, it is essential to treat everybody with respect and contribute to an atmosphere of dignity for all.
    - » For example, helpers involved in dead body management must treat the deceased person with dignity during the burial and ensure respect for their surviving family members.

Rights

- » Make sure people can access help fairly and without discrimination.
- » Help people to claim their rights and access available support.
- » Act only in the best interest of any person you encounter.

Keep these principles in mind in all of your actions and with all people you encounter, whatever their age, gender or ethnic background. Consider how you would like to be treated in that situation, and treat people in the same way.

Do's ✓

- » Be honest and trustworthy.
- » Respect people's right to make their own well-informed decisions.
- » Be aware of and set aside your own biases and prejudices.
- » Make it clear to people that even if they refuse help now, they can still access help in the future.
- » Respect privacy and keep personal details of the person's story confidential, if this is appropriate.
- » Behave appropriately by considering the person's culture, age and gender.

Don'ts ✗

- » Don't exploit your relationship as a helper.
- » Don't ask the person for any money or favour for helping.
- » Don't make false promises or give false information.
- » Don't exaggerate your skills.
- » Don't force help on people, and don't be intrusive or pushy.
- » Don't pressure people to tell you their story.
- » Don't share personal details of the person's story with others.
- » Don't judge the person for their actions or feelings.

2.2 BE AWARE OF OTHER AVAILABLE EMERGENCY RESPONSE MEASURES

An important part of offering PFA is to ensure that people have access to the correct information about Ebola, including what services and supports are available, and how to protect themselves. This also involves dispelling the many myths that often arise during frightening disease outbreaks.

Therefore, when offering PFA, it is essential to be aware of what other agencies are doing, and where and how people who may have the disease should seek help (e.g., know the contact information for key service providers). It is also important to know and share information about who is responsible for child protection, case management, food distribution and health care for people requiring treatment for illnesses other than Ebola.

2.3 LOOK AFTER YOURSELF

Helping responsibly means looking after your own physical and mental wellbeing.

As a helper, you may also be affected by the Ebola outbreak or may have family, friends and colleagues who are affected. It is essential to pay extra attention to your own wellbeing and be sure that you are physically and emotionally able to help others. **Take care of yourself first**, so that you can best care for others. If working in a team, also be aware of the wellbeing of your fellow helpers, and find ways to support each other.

> **As a helper, if you begin to exhibit any symptoms of the disease, <u>do not go to work</u>, as you will risk spreading the disease to co-workers and the people you are trying to help. Immediately inform your agency, seek medical care and take all necessary safety precautions to prevent infecting others.**

See Chapter 4 for more information on looking after yourself and your colleagues.

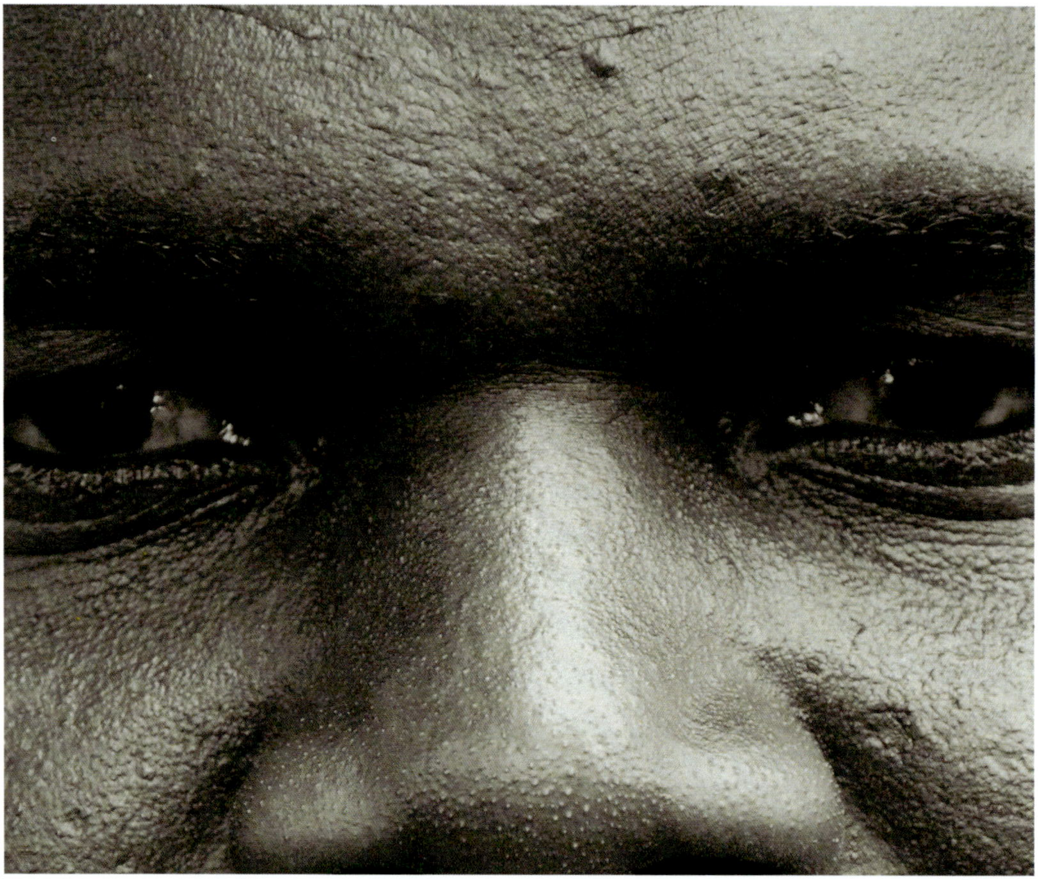

CHAPTER 3
PROVIDING PSYCHOLOGICAL FIRST AID

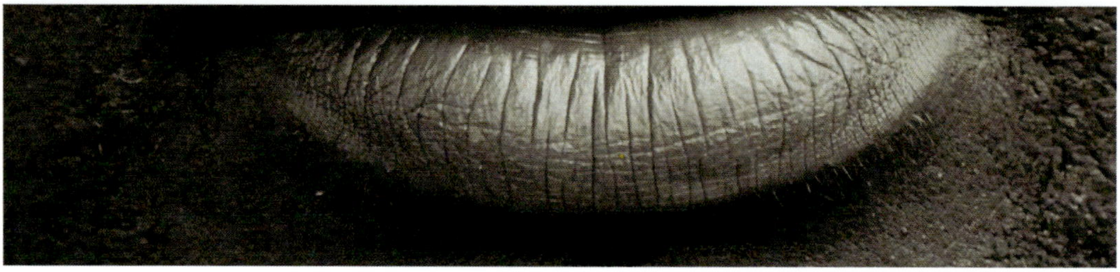

IN PROVIDING PFA, CONSIDER THE FOLLOWING:

3.1 GOOD COMMUNICATION WITH PEOPLE IN DISTRESS
3.2 PREPARING TO HELP
3.3 PFA ACTION PRINCIPLES: LOOK, LISTEN AND LINK!
3.4 HELPING PEOPLE WHO ARE LIKELY TO NEED SPECIAL ATTENTION

3.1 GOOD COMMUNICATION WITH PEOPLE IN DISTRESS

The way you communicate with someone in distress is very important. People who have been through a crisis event may be very upset, anxious or confused. Some people may blame themselves for things that happened and others may be angry, especially if they are grieving.

Being calm and showing understanding can help people in distress feel more safe and secure, understood, respected and cared for appropriately.

Someone who has been through a distressing event may want to tell you their story. Listening to someone's story can be a great support.

However, it is important not to pressure anyone to tell you what they have been through. Some people may not want to speak about what has happened or their circumstances. Nevertheless, they may value having you stay with them quietly, knowing you are there if they want to talk, or being offered practical support like a meal or a glass of water.

Don't talk too much. Keeping silent for a while may give the person space and encourage them to share with you if they wish.

To communicate well, be aware of both your words and body language, such as facial expressions, eye contact, gestures, and the way you sit or stand in relation to the other person. Speak and behave in ways that take into account the person's culture, age, gender, customs and religion.

Culture determines how we relate to people, and what is all right and not all right to say and do. For example, some people may not be used to sharing their feelings with someone outside of their family, or it may be appropriate for women to speak only with other women. You may be helping people from a different cultural background, or from a minority group, or someone who may be marginalized. **As a helper, it is important to**

be aware of your own cultural background and beliefs, so you can set aside your biases. Offer help in ways that are most appropriate and comfortable to the people you are supporting.

Below are suggestions for things to say and do, and what not to say and do. Most importantly, be yourself, be genuine and be sincere in offering your help and care.

THINGS TO SAY AND DO ✓	THINGS **NOT** TO SAY AND DO ✗
» Try to find a quiet place to talk, and minimize outside distractions. » Respect privacy and keep personal details of the person's story confidential, if this is appropriate. » Keep an appropriate distance from the person, depending on their age, gender and culture. » Let them know you are listening; for example, nod your head or say "hmmmm…." » Be patient and calm. » Provide factual information, if you have it. Be honest about what you know and don't know. "I don't know, but I will try to find out about that for you." » Give information in a way that any person can understand – keep it simple. » Acknowledge how they are feeling and any losses or important events they tell you about, such as the loss of their loved ones. "I'm so sorry. I can imagine this is very sad for you." » Acknowledge the person's strengths and how they have helped themselves. » Allow for silence.	» Don't pressure someone to tell their story (for example, don't look at your watch or speak too rapidly). » Don't touch the person and/or their body fluids, given the infectious nature of Ebola disease. » Don't judge what they have or haven't done, or how they are feeling. Don't say: "You shouldn't feel that way," or "You should feel lucky you survived." » Don't make up things you don't know. » Don't use terms that are too technical. » Don't tell them someone else's story. » Don't talk about your own troubles. » Don't give false promises or false reassurances. » Don't think and act as if you must solve all the person's problems for them. » Don't take away the person's strength and sense of being able to care for themselves. » Don't talk about people in negative terms (for example, don't call them "crazy" or "mad").

3.2 PREPARING TO HELP

Learn about Ebola disease from reliable resources – how it is transmitted, why it is so dangerous and the risks, signs and symptoms. (See Introduction)

Know what other agencies in the area are doing and where people can go to obtain more information about Ebola, or to talk to someone. Be aware of the procedures for referring people for immediate medical attention, and where and how people can access other support services.

For people who extra need help in coping emotionally and socially with the situation, know the contact information for relevant mental health and psychosocial resources in your area **(see CONTACT LIST OF MENTAL HEALTH AND PSYCHOSOCIAL RESOURCES IN YOUR AREA, page 54)**.

3.3 THE ACTION PRINCIPLES OF PFA: LOOK, LISTEN AND LINK!

LOOK
- » Check for safety.
- » Check for people with obvious urgent basic needs.
- » Check for people with serious distress reactions.

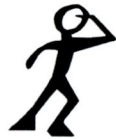

LISTEN
- » Approach people who may need support.
- » Ask about people's needs and concerns.
- » Listen to people, and help them to feel calm.

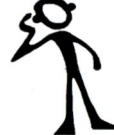

LINK
- » Help people address basic needs and access services.
- » Help people cope with problems.
- » Give information.
- » Connect people with loved ones and social support.

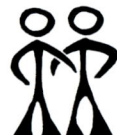

LOOK
- » Check for safety.
- » Check for people with obvious urgent basic needs.
- » Check for people with serious distress reactions.

Take time - even a few moments - to "look" around you before offering help. These moments will give you a chance to be calm, be safe and think before you act. See the following table for questions to consider and important messages as you "look" around you.

LOOK	QUESTIONS	IMPORTANT MESSAGE
Safety	» What dangers can you see in the environment? » Can you be there without likely harm to yourself or others?	If you are not certain about the health condition of the person you are talking to, **take all necessary safety precautions to protect yourself and others from infection**. Do not make physical contact with the person or their body fluids or tissues, or other potentially contaminated objects such as their clothing or bedding. Let the person know that you are physically healthy at present and that it is important for you to take precautions to prevent infection.
People with obvious urgent basic needs	» Does anyone appear to have symptoms of Ebola? » Who is most at risk in your area? » Does anybody have obvious urgent basic needs, such as clothing or food? » Who may need help to be protected from discrimination and violence?	Know your role and try to get help for people who need special assistance, such as those with obvious urgent basic needs. If the person has been exposed to the disease and/or has symptoms, encourage them to go to a treatment centre, local health post or Ebola Care Centre. If they cannot go to a health facility, immediately speak with your community leader or seek help from appropriately trained health care workers.
People in serious distress	» Are there people who appear extremely upset, in shock, not able to move on their own, or are not responding to others? » Where and who are the most distressed people?	Consider who may benefit from PFA and how you can best help.

Psychological first aid during Ebola virus disease outbreaks

People may react in various ways to a crisis event. Examples of psychological distress responses include:

- physical symptoms (shaking, headaches, tiredness, loss of appetite, aches and pains that have a non-medical basis). If there is no fever, these symptoms do not indicate Ebola;
- crying, sadness, depression and grief;
- anxiety and fear;
- being "on guard" or "jumpy";
- worrying that something bad is going to happen;
- insomnia and nightmares;
- irritability and anger;
- guilt and shame (for surviving, infecting others, or for not being able to help or save others);
- confusion, emotional numbness, or feeling unreal or in a daze;
- appearing withdrawn or very still (not moving);
- not responding to others, or not speaking at all;
- disorientation (not knowing their own name, where they are from, or what happened);
- not being able to care for themselves or their children (not eating or drinking, not able to make simple decisions).

Some people may be only mildly distressed or not distressed at all.

Most people will recover emotionally over time, especially if they receive support from others and help in meeting their basic needs. However, **people with severe and/or long-lasting distress may need more support than PFA**, particularly if they cannot function in their daily life or if they are a danger to themselves or others. Ensure that severely distressed people are not left alone and try to keep them safe until you can contact the relevant mental health and psychosocial support resources in your area **(see CONTACT LIST OF MENTAL HEALTH AND PSYCHOSOCIAL RESOURCES IN YOUR AREA, page 54)**.

Vulnerable People
Remember to look for children, people with other health conditions or physical and mental disabilities, and people at risk of discrimination, as they are likely to need special attention for their care and safety.

LISTEN
- » Approach people who may need support.
- » Ask about people's needs and concerns.
- » Listen to people, and help them to feel calm.

Listening carefully to a person you are helping is essential to understand their situation and needs, to help them feel calm, and to offer them appropriate help. Learn to listen with your:

- » Eyes » giving the person your undivided attention;
- » Ears » truly hearing their concerns;
- » Heart » with care and showing respect.

Even if you must communicate from a distance because of safety precautions, you can still give the person your full attention and show that you are listening with care.

1. APPROACH PEOPLE WHO MAY NEED SUPPORT:

- » Approach people respectfully, keeping a safe distance.
- » Introduce yourself by name and organization.
- » Explain that **while you can't touch them, you can listen and care about how they are feeling**. Ask the person how he/she is feeling and coping with the situation, and if you can provide help.
- » Be sure to ask about the person's physical condition, and let them know that you are physically healthy at present.
- » If possible, find a safe and quiet place to talk.
- » Ensure that the person is not putting others at risk of infection.
- » If the person is very distressed, try to ensure they are not alone until further help can be found.

2. ASK ABOUT PEOPLE'S NEEDS AND CONCERNS:

- » Although some needs may be obvious, such as some rest for a nurse who has been working long hours in the treatment centre, always ask what people need and what their concerns are.
- » Find out what is most important to them at this moment, and help them work out what their priorities are.
- » Ask whether they need anything that can be provided to them from a safe distance (e.g., fresh water, food, clean clothes or bedding).

3. LISTEN TO PEOPLE AND HELP THEM TO FEEL CALM:

- » Do not pressure the person to talk.
- » Listen in case they want to talk about what happened.
- » Offer to sing, read, or tell stories to reassure them they are not alone and ease their fear.
- » If they are very distressed, help them to feel calm and try to ensure they are not left alone.

HELP PEOPLE TO FEEL CALM

Some people in a crisis situation may be very anxious or upset. They may feel confused or overwhelmed, and may have physical reactions such as shaking or trembling, difficulty breathing, or feeling that their heart is pounding. The following are some techniques to help very distressed people feel calm in their mind and body:

- Keep your tone of voice calm and soft.
- Try to maintain some eye contact with the person as you talk with them.
- Remind the person that you are there to help them. Remind them that they are safe, if it is true.
- If someone feels unreal or disconnected from their surroundings, it may help them to make contact with their current environment and themselves. You can do this by asking them to:
    - Place and feel their feet on the floor.
    - Tap their fingers or hands on their lap.
    - Notice some non-distressing things in their environment, such as things they can see, hear or feel. Have them tell you what they see and hear.
    - Encourage the person to focus on their breathing, and to breathe slowly.

LINK

» Help people address basic needs and access services.
» Help people cope with problems.
» Give information.
» Connect people with loved ones and social support.

1. HELP PEOPLE ADDRESS BASIC NEEDS AND ACCESS SERVICES

People affected by an Ebola disease outbreak, such as those whose property was destroyed during disinfection of their home, may need help in addressing basic needs and accessing services. As you provide PFA, consider the following:

» Try to help the person in distress to meet the basic needs they request, such as food, water, shelter and information about medical and social services.
» Learn what specific needs people have and try to link them to the help available (e.g., survival kits if their property was destroyed).
» Ensure vulnerable and marginalized people are not overlooked (see Section 3.4).
» Follow up with people if you promise to do so.

2. HELP PEOPLE COPE WITH PROBLEMS

A person in distress can feel overwhelmed with worries and fears. Help them to consider their most urgent needs, and how to prioritize and address them. For example, you can ask them to think about what they need to address now, and what can wait for later. Being able to manage a few issues will give the person a greater sense of control and strengthen their ability to cope.

Remember to:

- help people identify supports in their life, such as friends or family, who can help them. If they have lost many relatives and friends to Ebola, help them to think of additional supports, such as religious leaders or other members of the community;
- give practical suggestions for people to meet their own needs;
- ask the person to consider how they have coped with difficult situations in the past, and affirm their ability to cope with the current situation;
- ask the person what helps them to feel better. Encourage them to use positive coping strategies and avoid negative coping strategies (see the following table).

COPING

Everyone has natural ways of coping. Encourage people to use their own positive coping strategies, while avoiding negative strategies. This will help them to feel stronger and to regain a sense of control. You will need to adapt the following suggestions to take into account the person's culture and what is possible in the particular crisis situation.

Encourage positive coping strategies	<ul><li>Get enough rest.</li><li>Eat as regularly as possible and drink water.</li><li>Talk and spend time with family, friends or other community members.</li><li>Discuss problems with someone you trust.</li><li>Do activities that help you relax (walk, sing, pray).</li><li>Do physical exercise.</li><li>Find safe ways to help others in the crisis and get involved in community activities.</li></ul>
Discourage negative coping strategies	<ul><li>Don't take drugs, smoke or drink alcohol.</li><li>Don't sleep all day.</li><li>Don't work all the time without any rest or relaxation.</li><li>Don't isolate yourself from friends and loved ones.</li><li>Don't neglect basic personal hygiene.</li><li>Don't be violent.</li></ul>

3. GIVE INFORMATION

People affected by the outbreak will want accurate information about:

- Ebola virus disease
  - See facts about Ebola **in the introduction**.
  - Try to keep yourself informed of the latest updates on the outbreak.
- Loved ones
  - Try to share practical information with the relatives of patients in treatment centres. This should be done in consultation with staff, to ensure the information shared is appropriate, does not breach confidentiality and does not cause confusion by giving conflicting messages.
  - Try to find ways that family members can maintain contact with the patient. For example, relatives could give health workers items or messages of love and encouragement to pass on to the patient.
- Their safety
  - Share information about how to stay safe.
  - Share information about measures the government is taking to support victims during and after the outbreak.
- Their rights and responsibilities
  - This includes their rights to treatment and care, legal rights, being treated with dignity, etc.
  - This also includes their responsibility to follow the guidance of local authorities and health workers.
- Services and supports
  - This includes how to access services and other things they need.

Getting accurate information during the outbreak may be difficult. The situation may change as information about the number of cases, areas affected, etc., becomes known and relief measures are put in place.

Rumours may be common

The less information that is shared, the more likely it is that rumours will spread. Sharing accurate information is the best way to stop rumours. Try to be aware of the more common rumours so that you are prepared to respond with reliable and accurate information. Rumours may be very dangerous; for example, rumours that blame certain people for the disease outbreak may lead to violence, or rumours about fake, harmful treatments may lead to unnecessary deaths.

You may not have all the answers at any given moment, but wherever possible, try to get as much information as you can before you offer people support and information. It may be helpful to use official written information, such as posters and leaflets in the local language, or in pictorial form for people with low literacy, to complement the information you are giving. Try to ensure vulnerable people know about existing services and how to obtain information (see Section 3.4).

When providing information:

- » explain the source of the information and how reliable it is;
- » say only what you know – do not make up information or give false reassurances;
- » keep messages simple and accurate, and repeat the information to be sure people hear and understand it;
- » it may be useful to give information to groups of affected people, so that everyone hears the same message;
- » let people know if you will keep them updated on new developments, including where and when.

When giving information, be aware that the helper can become a target of the frustration and anger people may feel, especially when their expectations of help have not been met by you or others. In these situations, try to remain calm and be understanding.

4. CONNECT WITH LOVED ONES AND SOCIAL SUPPORT

It has been shown that people who feel they had good social support after a crisis cope better than those who feel they were not well supported. Because of this, linking people with loved ones and social support is an important part of PFA.

This task may be very difficult, as many people may have lost most of their loved ones to Ebola, and because of the stigma associated with the illness. Affected people can feel very isolated. Therefore, it will be very important to help people identify who else within their community could be of support. There may be existing groups and community networks that can provide support.

Mental health and psychosocial workers can help those lacking social support by visiting or accompanying them. Social reintegration in the community for those who survived Ebola or those confirmed negative for the disease is also important. This can help to reduce stigma, decrease other people's fear of interacting with them, and to identify other sources of support if relatives are missing.

In connecting people with loved ones and social support:

- » Help keep families together, and keep children with their parents and loved ones if possible, while also observing the safety measures to avoid Ebola disease transmission. If a child with Ebola is admitted to hospital, they should be able to have safe and regular contact with one trusted family member.
    - » *Refer to the information on **People who likely need special attention** in Section 3.4 regarding the specific needs of children and adolescents that have lost parents to Ebola or are being rejected in their communities.*
- » Help people to contact friends and relatives so they can get support; for example, provide a way for them to call loved ones, including admitted patients.
    - » *Use **phones to give psychosocial support**: a phone could be made available at the treatment centre for patients' use only, so relatives can talk to their loved ones.*

- » If a person lets you know that prayer, religious practice or support from religious leaders might be helpful for them, try to connect them with their spiritual community, always observing safety measures.
  - » *Given the risk of spreading the disease in public gatherings or through direct contact, it is important to find new ways of praying together. For example, relatives or religious leaders could pray with patients in treatment centres through the telephone, or possibly from across the safety barrier of dedicated disease centres, if they are permitted. Religious leaders can also help by finding new ways to provide spiritual support and guidance that don't involve touching to prevent the spread of disease and to protect people by preventing the spread of disease.*

- » Help bring affected people together to support each other. For example, ask people to help care for the elderly or the children who have lost their carers, or link individuals without family to other community members.
  - » *See the section on **Offering PFA to grieving people** to help affected families and communities who cannot engage in traditional burials (due to the risk of spreading the disease) to find new ways of mourning and honouring the deceased.*

Ending Your Help

What happens next? When and how you stop providing help to someone will depend on the situation of the Ebola disease outbreak, your role and circumstances, and the needs of the person you are helping. You may be working in the affected community for some time, but if you are ending your assistance with someone, explain that you are leaving. If someone else will be helping the person after you, try to introduce them. If you have linked the person with other services, let them know what to expect and be sure they have the details to follow up. No matter what your experience with the person, you can say goodbye in a positive way by wishing them well.

3.4 PEOPLE WHO LIKELY NEED SPECIAL ATTENTION

People who may be vulnerable and need special help in a crisis include:

1. Children, including adolescents.

2. People with health conditions or disabilities.

3. People at risk of discrimination or violence.

Remember that all people have resources to cope, including those who are vulnerable. Help vulnerable people to use their own coping resources and strategies.

1. CHILDREN, INCLUDING ADOLESCENTS

Children with suspected Ebola should always be accompanied to a hospital, local health post or designated Ebola Care Centre.

If a parent needs medical attention, consideration must be taken to ensure any children in their care will be looked after and not left to fend for themselves.

Many children – including adolescents – are particularly vulnerable in an outbreak. Ebola disease disrupts their familiar world, including the people, places and routines that make them feel secure. Many will have lost their parents and other relatives. There are reports of children being abandoned. Stigma and discrimination is isolating them from protection and support, and putting them at a great risk. Young children are particularly vulnerable since they cannot meet their own basic needs or protect themselves. Girls usually face the greatest risk of sexual violence and exploitation, and those who have been abused may be stigmatized and further isolated. Girls and young women can be at greater risk of exposure to Ebola disease, when they are caregivers or frontline health staff.

How children react to a crisis depends on their age and developmental stage. It also depends on the ways their carers and other adults interact with them. For example, young children may not fully understand what is happening around them, and are especially in need of support.

Children generally cope better when they have a stable, calm adult around them.

Children and young people may experience similar distress reactions as adults (see Section 3.3). They may also experience the following specific distress reactions:

- Young children may return to earlier behaviours (for example, bedwetting or thumb-sucking), cling to carers, and reduce their play or use repetitive play related to the distressing event.
- School-age children may believe they caused bad things to happen, develop new fears, become less affectionate, feel alone and be preoccupied with protecting or rescuing people in the crisis.
- Adolescents may feel "nothing", feel different or isolated from their friends, or display risk-taking behaviour and negative attitudes.

Family and other caregivers are important sources of protection and emotional support for children. Those separated from caregivers (e.g., orphans because of Ebola) may find themselves in unfamiliar places and around unfamiliar people during an Ebola disease outbreak. They may be very fearful and may not be able to properly judge the risks and danger around them.

An important first step is to reunite separated children – including adolescents – with their families or carers. If this is not possible (e.g., family or carers are deceased), try to link them immediately with a trustworthy child protection agency (governmental or non-governmental) that can begin the process of registering the child and ensuring they are cared for. The agency may be able to reunite them with relatives in other areas, or with other trusted members of the community that they know, such as neighbours or distant relatives.

It is very important not to do this on your own, but rather to work through child protection agencies. If you make mistakes, it will make the child's situation worse **(see CONTACT LIST OF EBOLA DISEASE OUTBREAK SERVICES IN YOUR AREA, back cover).**

Children may witness horrific events, even if they or their carers are not directly affected. For example, they might be curious about the health workers wearing protective clothing, follow them, and witness how they take a person in an advanced state of the disease from their home. Or they may see people who have died of the disease. In the chaos of a crisis, adults are often busy and may not be watching closely what children are doing or what they see or hear. Try to shield them from upsetting scenes or stories.

Remember that children have their own resources for coping.

Learn what children's resources are for coping and support positive coping strategies, while helping them to avoid negative strategies. Older children and adolescents can often help in crisis situations, such as putting up posters with accurate information about Ebola. Finding safe ways for them to contribute may help them to feel more in control. Children, adolescents and youth may also have networks and associations that can provide social support.

HOW CARERS CAN HELP CHILDREN

Infants	
»	Keep them warm and safe.
»	Keep them away from loud noises and chaos.
»	Keep a regular feeding and sleeping schedule, if possible.
»	Speak in a calm and soft voice.

Young children	
»	Give them extra time and attention.
»	Remind them often that they are safe.
»	Explain to them that they are not to blame for bad things that have happened.
»	Whenever possible, avoid separating young children from parents and carers, siblings, and other loved ones.
»	Keep to regular routines and schedules as much as possible, or help create new ones in a new environment.
»	Give simple answers about what has happened without scary details.
»	Allow them to stay close to you if they are fearful or clingy.
»	Be patient with children who start demonstrating behaviours they had when they were younger, such as sucking their thumb or wetting the bed.
»	Provide a chance to play and relax, if possible.

HOW CARERS CAN HELP CHILDREN (continued)

Older children and adolescents

- » Give them your time and attention.
- » Help them to keep regular routines, including school/learning.
- » Provide facts about what has happened, explain what is going on now and give them clear information about how to reduce their risk of being infected by the disease.
- » Encourage and allow opportunities for them to be helpful in concrete, purposeful common interests (e.g., taking on safe but relevant tasks in the community as part of the overall outbreak response).
- » Allow them to be sad. Don't expect them to be tough.
- » Listen to their thoughts and fears without being judgemental.
- » Set clear rules and expectations.
- » Ask them about the dangers they face, support them and discuss how they can best avoid being harmed.
- » Link them with existing networks of adolescents, youth and other community and social support groups.

When providing PFA to children, remember to **Listen, Talk and Play**:

- » Be calm, talk softly and be kind.
- » Listen to children's views on their situation.
- » Try to talk with them at their eye level (e.g. sit or kneel on the floor), and use words and explanations they can understand.
- » Introduce yourself by name, let them know you are healthy and that you are there to help.
- » If talking with a child who has Ebola, explain that *although you can't touch them, you can listen and care about how they are feeling*.
- » Find out their name, where they are from, and any information you can in order to help find their caregivers and other family members.
- » If passing time with children, try to involve them in play activities or simple conversation about their interests, according to their age and to the safety regulations for Ebola.

CHAPTER 3

2. PEOPLE WITH HEALTH CONDITIONS OR PHYSICAL OR MENTAL DISABILITIES

People with chronic (long-term) health conditions, with physical or mental disabilities (including severe mental disorder), and the elderly may need special help. This may include help to get to a safe place, to connect with basic support and health care, or to take care of themselves. The experience of a crisis event, and the impact of Ebola disease on the availability of medical resources, can worsen different types of health conditions, such as high blood pressure, heart conditions, asthma, anxiety and other health and mental disorders. Pregnant and nursing women may experience severe stress from the crisis that can affect their pregnancy, their own health and their infant's health. People who cannot move on their own, or who have problems seeing or hearing, may have difficulty finding loved ones or accessing services.

Here are some things you can do to help people with other health conditions or disabilities:

- » Help them to get to a safe place.
- » Help them to meet their basic needs, such as being able to eat, drink, get clean water and care for themselves.
- » Ask people if they have any health conditions other than Ebola, or if they regularly take medication for a health problem. Try to help people get their medication or access available medical services.
- » Stay with the person if they are very distressed, or try to ensure they have someone to help them if you need to leave. Consider linking the person with a protection agency or other relevant support, to help them in the longer term.
- » Help them if they are experiencing Ebola disease symptoms. Avoid physical contact, but help refer them for immediate medical care. Ensure other people do not come into contact with them.

3. PEOPLE AT RISK OF DISCRIMINATION OR VIOLENCE

People at risk of discrimination or violence may include women, people from certain ethnic or religious groups, and people with mental and physical disabilities. In the case of an Ebola disease outbreak, people at risk may include relatives of those affected by Ebola, relatives wanting to bury the dead, and people working in Ebola operations (e.g., people doing contact tracing or dead body management). They are vulnerable because they may be:

- left out when basic services are provided;
- left out of decisions about aid, services or where to go; and
- targeted for violence, including sexual violence.

People at risk of discrimination or violence may need special protection to be safe in a crisis situation, and may need extra help to address their basic needs and access available services. Be aware of these people and assist them by:

- helping them to find safe places to stay;
- helping them to connect with their loved ones and other trusted people;
- providing them with information on available services and helping them to link directly with those services when necessary.
- As above, help them if they are experiencing Ebola disease symptoms. Do not have physical contact with them if you don't have the necessary equipment for your protection, but help refer them for immediate medical care.

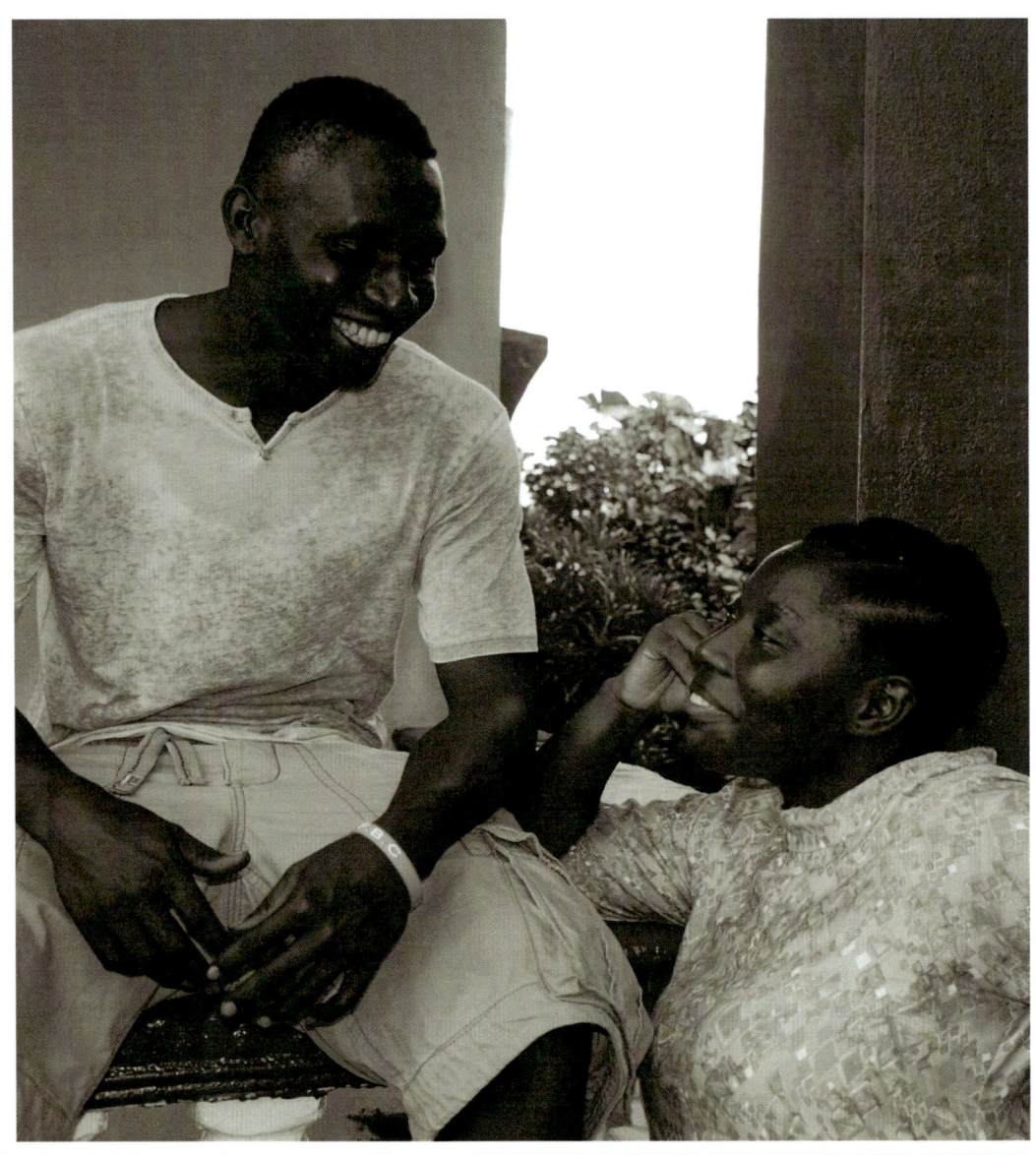

CHAPTER 4
CARING FOR YOURSELF AND YOUR COLLEAGUES

IN THIS CHAPTER, WE WILL DISCUSS:

4.1 GETTING READY TO HELP
4.2 MANAGING STRESS: HEALTHY WORK AND LIFE HABITS
4.3 REST AND REFLECTION

You or your family may be directly affected by the Ebola outbreak. Even if you are not directly involved, you may be affected by what you see or hear while helping. As a helper, it is important to **pay extra attention to your own wellbeing**. Take care of yourself, so you can best take care of others!

4.1 GETTING READY TO HELP

Consider how you can best get ready to be a helper in crisis settings. Whenever possible:

» Learn about the Ebola disease outbreak situation, and the roles and responsibilities of different kinds of helpers (e.g., health authorities and community workers).
» Consider your own health, and personal or family issues that may cause severe stress as you take on a helping role for others.
» Make an honest decision about whether you are ready to help in each particular situation and at this particular time.
» Be sure that you know and understand how to observe all the safety measures to avoid Ebola disease.

4.2 MANAGING STRESS: HEALTHY WORK AND LIFE HABITS

A main source of stress for helpers is day-to-day job stress, particularly during a disease outbreak. Long working hours, overwhelming responsibilities, the lack of a clear job description, poor communication or management, and working in areas that are not secure are examples of common job-related stress that can affect helpers assisting in the outbreak.

As a helper, you may feel responsible for people's safety and care. You may witness or even directly experience terrible things, such as death, severe illness and suffering, social unrest or violence. You may also hear stories of other people's pain and suffering. All of these experiences can affect you and your fellow helpers.

Consider how you can best manage your own stress, to support and be supported by your fellow helpers. The following suggestions may be helpful in managing your stress:

- » Think about what has helped you cope in the past and what you can do to stay strong.
- » Try to take time to eat, rest and relax, even for short periods.
- » Try to keep reasonable working hours so you do not become too exhausted. Consider, for example, dividing the workload among helpers, working in shifts during the acute phase of the crisis and taking regular rest periods.
- » You may feel inadequate or frustrated when you cannot help people with all of their problems. Remember that you are not responsible for solving all of a person's problems, and it is not realistic or possible for you to do so. Do what you can to help people help themselves.
- » Minimize your intake of alcohol, caffeine or nicotine and avoid non-prescription drugs.
- » Check in with fellow helpers to see how they are doing, and have them check in with you. Find ways to support each other.
- » Talk with friends, loved ones or other people you trust for support.

4.3 REST AND REFLECTION

Taking time for rest and reflection is an important part of ending your helping role. The Ebola crisis situation and the needs of people you have met may have been very challenging, and it can be difficult to bear their pain and suffering. After helping in the outbreak, take time to reflect on your experience and to rest. The following suggestions may help your recovery:

- » Talk about your experience of helping in the crisis situation with a supervisor, colleague or someone else you trust.
- » Acknowledge what you were able to do to help others, even in small ways.
- » Learn to reflect on and accept what you did well, what did not go very well, and the limits of what you could do in the circumstances.
- » Take some time, if possible, to rest and relax before beginning your work and life duties again.

If you find yourself with upsetting thoughts or memories about the event, feel very nervous or extremely sad, have trouble sleeping, or drink a lot of alcohol or take drugs, it is important to get support from someone you trust. Speak to a mental health specialist if these difficulties continue for more than one month **(see CONTACT LIST OF MENTAL HEALTH AND PSYCHOSOCIAL RESOURCES IN YOUR AREA, page 54)**.

OFFERING PSYCHOLOGICAL FIRST AID TO GRIEVING PEOPLE

In many crisis situations the normal rituals and processes that help people grieve and say goodbye to their loved ones cannot occur. This is particularly true in the case of Ebola disease. For example, local cultural or religious practices for burials may not be possible because of the risk of spreading infection.

Losing a loved one can be like a wound that hurts. It can leave people feeling very angry and frustrated that they do not have a way to honour and remember their loved ones. People may feel overwhelmed with sadness because of their loss and the situation they are in. They may be unable to accept that the person has died. These are all normal grief reactions following the loss of a loved one.

It is important to recognise that people need the time and space to grieve. In many cultures, traditional and religious rituals and burial ceremonies enable the person or family to start coping with their loss of a loved one. Not being able to engage in these ceremonies because of the risk of disease spread may create more anger, sadness and fear.

It is essential to inform grieving people about the risks and dangers of handling the body of a person who has died of Ebola, but also reassure them that there can be other ways of grieving, honouring and remembering the person.

If you are offering PFA to bereaved people it is important to:

» Help them feel calm and safe.
» Listen to them and allow them the time and space to feel sad and grieve.
» If they wish, you can introduce them to others who have been bereaved and encourage them to support each other.
» Allow them the time and space to talk about their loved ones.
» If they are struggling to accept that they cannot bury their loved ones in a traditional ceremony, encourage them to think of alternative ways that they can honour, remember and grieve for them.
» Consider engaging religious leaders in helping to develop alternative rituals that are safe for the mourners (see Annex for space to record local alternative rituals for safe mourning).

Ideas for safely mourning and honouring the deceased:

People affected by Ebola disease have come up with new ways that help people to grieve, without engaging in traditional ceremonies and rituals that involve handling the dead body:

» In other cultures, individuals and families have planted trees in remembrance of their loved ones.
» Others have been able to hold memorial services for their loved ones using photographs of the person as a focal point.

It may be helpful to share these ideas with bereaved families and communities, and help them consider ways of safely mourning their loved ones that will work for them.

RELAXATION AND BREATHING EXERCISES

Relaxation is a useful way of reducing stress, and deep breathing helps the body and mind to relax so that people can stay healthy and calm. Many traditional types of meditation as well as modern psychology use some form of breathing exercise to teach people how to relax.

However, before you can teach others, you should try it yourself. Try following the steps below to experience the sense of relaxation it can give. Then you can instruct others in the exercise using the instructions below. Remember to speak slowly and in a calm tone of voice.

RELAXATION EXERCISE SCRIPT

During stressful times, it is important to find ways to relax the mind and body so that we can cope effectively with challenges, demands and emotions. Deep breathing helps to trigger relaxation to help people stay healthy and calm during difficult times. By practising this EVERY day for a few weeks, most people will start to feel more relaxed and better able to cope.

You can do the following exercise at any time of the day. Try to devote at least 5 minutes a day to the exercise. It is best done in a quiet room where you will not be disturbed.

Let us practise together:

- Begin by lying down or sitting in a comfortable position. There is no special position, just find a position that feels comfortable for you.
- Close your eyes and relax your face. Feel yourself supported by your chair or by the floor if you are lying down. Begin to relax any tension you feel in your body.
- Begin to concentrate on the rhythm of your breath. Slowly feel your breath as you inhale through your nose, and then as you exhale through your nose. Feel the air filling your lungs and circulating through the body with each inhale and exhale.
- Now, inhale slowly to the count of four *(count slowly with the person to the pace of one-one-thousand, two-one-thousand....)*. Pause with the breath held in to the count of three. Then, exhale slowly to the count of five.
    - *Continue with this breathing process for a few minutes, instructing the person to breathe regularly and slowly like this:*

        Inhale... two, three, four...Pause...two, three....Exhale...two, three, four, five....
        Inhale... two, three, four...Pause...two, three....Exhale...two, three, four, five....

- *You can suggest that each time they breathe out they say in their mind the word 'relax' or an equivalent in their local language. People who are religious may want to say a word that is important to their faith.*
- To end the exercise, feel the relaxation you have created in your body and mind. Thank yourself for this important time of rest and care.

CONTACT LIST OF MENTAL HEALTH AND PSYCHOSOCIAL RESOURCES IN YOUR AREA

	Name	Contact	Type of Service Provided	Notes
1				
2				
3				
4				
5				
6				
7				
8				
9				
10				

LOCAL ALTERNATIVE RITUALS FOR SAFE MOURNING AFTER THE DEATH OF A PERSON WITH EBOLA

1.
2.
3.
4.
5.
6.

Psychological first aid: Pocket guide

WHAT IS PSYCHOLOGICAL FIRST AID?

Psychological First Aid (PFA) describes a humane, supportive response to a person who is suffering and may need support.

Providing PFA responsibly means:
1. Respecting people's safety, dignity and rights.
2. Adapting what you do to take into account the person's culture.
3. Being aware of other emergency response measures.
4. Looking after yourself.

In providing PFA responsibly during an Ebola virus disease outbreak:

» Ensure people know their rights (such as right to treatment and care, being treated with dignity, etc.) *as well as their responsibilities* in the Ebola disease outbreak, such as their responsibility to follow the guidance of local health authorities and health workers.

» Look after your own physical and mental wellbeing! As a helper, you may also be affected by the Ebola outbreak or may have family, friends and colleagues who are affected. Pay extra attention to your own wellbeing and be sure that you follow all safety precautions.

PREPARE
» Learn about Ebola virus disease.
» Learn about available services and supports.
» Learn about safety and security concerns.

PFA ACTION PRINCIPLES:

LOOK
» Check for safety.
» Check for people with obvious urgent basic needs.
» Check for people with serious distress reactions.

LISTEN
» Approach people who may need support.
» Ask about people's needs and concerns.
» Listen to people, and help them to feel calm.

Even if you must communicate from a distance because of safety precautions, you can still give the person your full attention and show that you are listening with care.

LINK
» Help people address basic needs and access services.
» Help people cope with problems.
» Give information.
» Connect people with loved ones and social support.

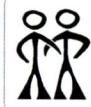

Psychological first aid during Ebola virus disease outbreaks